A Detailed Vegan Cookbook

Vegan Cookbook with Pictures,

Quickly and Healthy Meals,

Delicious Food to Change Your Life

Franck Renner

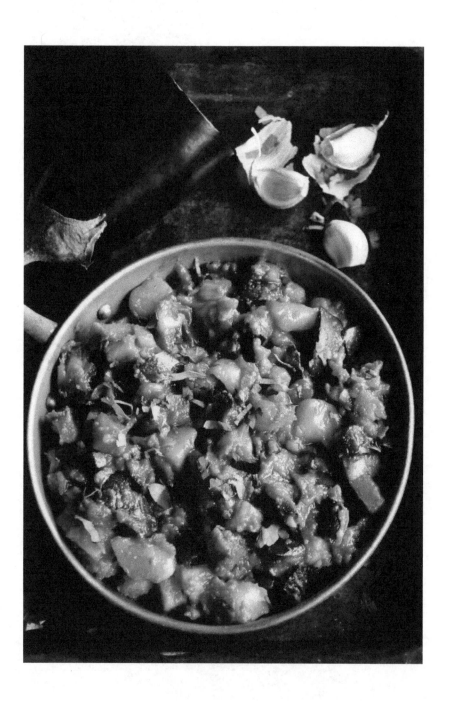

Table of Contents

secondary or tertiary copy of the work or a recorded copy and is only allowed with the express written consent from the Publisher. All additional right reserved.

The information in the following pages is broadly considered a truthful and accurate account of facts and as such, any inattention, use, or misuse of the information in question by the reader will render any resulting actions solely under their purview. There are no scenarios in which the publisher or the original author of this work can be in any fashion deemed liable for any hardship or damages that may befall them after undertaking information described herein.

Additionally, the information in the following pages is intended only for informational purposes and should thus be thought of as universal. As befitting its nature, it is presented without assurance regarding its prolonged validity or interim quality. Trademarks that are mentioned are done without

written consent and can in no way be considered an
endorsement from the trademark holder.

INTRODUCTION

The Merriam Webster Dictionary defines a vegetarian as one contains a wholly of vegetables, grains, nuts, fruits, and sometimes eggs or dairy products. It has also been described as a plant-based diet that relies wholly on plant-foods such as fruits, whole grains, herbs, vegetables, nuts, seeds, and spices. Whatever way you want to look at it, the reliance wholly on plants stands the vegetarian diet out from other types of diets. People become vegetarians for different reasons. Some take up this nutritional plan for medical or health reasons. For example, people suffering from cardiovascular diseases or who stand the risk of developing such diseases are usually advised to refrain from meat generally and focus on a plant-based diet, rich in fruits and vegetables. Some other individuals become vegetarians for religious or ethical reasons.

On this side of the spectrum are Hinduism, Jainism, Buddhism, Seventh-Day Adventists, and some other religions. It is believed that being a vegetarian is part of being holy and keeping with the ideals of non-violence. For ethical reasons, some animal rights activists are also vegetarians based on the belief that animals have rights and should not be slaughtered for food. Yet another set of persons become vegetarians based on food preference. Such individuals are naturally more disposed to a plant-based diet and find meat and other related food products less pleasurable. Some refrain from meat as a protest against climate change. This is based on the environmental concern that rearing livestock contributes to climate change and greenhouse gas emissions and the waste of natural resources in maintaining such livestock. People are usually very quick to throw words around without exactly knowing what a Vegetarian Diet means. In the same vein, the term "vegetarian" has become a popular one in recent years. What exactly does this word connote, and what does it not mean?

At its simplest, the word "vegetarian" refers to a person who refrains from eating meat, beef, pork, lard, chicken, or even fish. Depending on the kind of vegetarian it is, however, a vegetarian could either eat or exclude from his diet animal products. Animal products would refer to foods such as eggs, dairy products, and even honey! A vegetarian diet would, therefore, refer to the nutritional plan of the void of meat. It is the eating lifestyle of individuals who depend on plant-based foods for nutrition. It excludes animal products, particularly meat - a common denominator for all kinds of Vegetarians - from their diets. A vegetarian could also be defined as a meal plan that consists of foods coming majorly from plants to the exclusion of meat, poultry, and seafood.

This kind of Vegetarian diet usually contains no animal protein.

It is completely understandable from the discussion so far that the term "vegetarian" is more or less a blanket term covering different plant-based diets. While reliance majorly on plant foods is consistent in all the different types of vegetarians, they have some underlying differences. The different types of vegetarians are discussed below:

Veganism: This is undoubtedly the strictest type of vegetarian diet. Vegans exclude the any animal product. It goes as far as avoiding animal-derived ingredients contained in processed foods. Whether its meat, poultry products like eggs, dairy products inclusive of milk, honey, or even gelatin, they all are excluded from the vegans.

Some vegans go beyond nutrition and go as far as refusing to wear clothes that contain animal products. This means such vegans do not wear leather, wool, or silk.

Lacto-vegetarian: This kind of vegetarian excludes meat, fish, and poultry. However, it allows the inclusion of dairy products such as milk, yogurt, cheese, and butter. The hint is perhaps in the name since Lacto means milk in Latin.

Ovo-Vegetarian: Meat and dairy products are excluded under this diet, but eggs could be consumed. Ovo means egg.

Lacto-Ovo Vegetarian: This appears to be the hybrid of the Ovo Vegetarian and the Lacto-Vegetarian. This is the most famous type of vegetarian diet and is usually what comes to mind when people think of the Vegetarian. This type of Vegetarian bars all kinds of meat but allows for the consumption of eggs and dairy products.

Pollotarian: This vegetarian allows the consumption of chicken.

Pescatarian: This refers to the vegetarian that consumes fish. More people are beginning to subscribe to this kind of diet due to health reasons.

Flexitarian: Flexitarians are individuals who prefer plant-based foods to meat but have no problem eating meats once in a while. They are also referred to as semi-vegetarians.

Raw Vegan: This is also called the raw food and consists of a vegan that is yet to be processed and has also not been heated over 46 C. This kind of diet has its root in the belief that nutrients and minerals present in the plant diet are lost when cooked on temperature above 46 C and could also become harmful to the body.

Pear Lemonade

Preparation Time: 5 minutes

Cooking Time: 30 minutes

Servings: 2 servings

Ingredients:

- ½ cup of pear, peeled and diced
- 1 cup of freshly squeezed lemon juice
- ½ cup of chilled water

Directions:

1. Add all the ingredients into a blender and pulse until it has all been combined. The pear does make the lemonade frothy, but this will settle.
2. Place in the refrigerator to cool and then serve.

Tips:

Keep stored in a sealed container in the refrigerator for up to four days.

Pop the fresh lemon in the microwave for ten minutes before juicing, you can extract more juice if you do this.

Nutrition: Calories: 160 Carbs: 6.3g Protein: 2.9g

Fat: 13.6g

Energizing Ginger Detox Tonic

Preparation Time: 15 minutes

Cooking Time: 10 minutes

Servings:

Ingredients:

- 1/2 teaspoon of grated ginger, fresh
- 1 small lemon slice
- 1/8 teaspoon of cayenne pepper
- 1/8 teaspoon of ground turmeric
- 1/8 teaspoon of ground cinnamon
- 1 teaspoon of maple syrup
- 1 teaspoon of apple cider vinegar
- 2 cups of boiling water

Directions:

1. Pour the boiling water into a small saucepan, add and stir the ginger, then let it rest for 8 to 10 minutes, before covering the pan.
2. Pass the mixture through a strainer and into the liquid, add the cayenne pepper, turmeric, cinnamon and stir properly.
3. Add the maple syrup, vinegar, and lemon slice.

4. Add and stir an infused lemon and serve immediately.

Nutrition: Calories 443 Carbs: 9.7 g Protein: 62.8g Fat: 16.9g

Warm Spiced Lemon Drink

Preparation Time: 10 minutes

Cooking Time: 2 hours

Servings: 12

Ingredients:

- 1 cinnamon stick, about 3 inches long
- 1/2 teaspoon of whole cloves
- 2 cups of coconut sugar
- 4 fluid of ounce pineapple juice
- 1/2 cup and 2 tablespoons of lemon juice
- 12 fluid ounce of orange juice
- 2 1/2 quarts of water

Directions:

1. Pour water into a 6-quarts slow cooker and stir the sugar and lemon juice properly.
2. Wrap the cinnamon, the whole cloves in cheesecloth and tie its corners with string.
3. Immerse this cheesecloth bag in the liquid present in the slow cooker and cover it with the lid.

4. Then plug in the slow cooker and let it cook on high heat setting for 2 hours or until it is heated thoroughly.

5. When done, discard the cheesecloth bag and serve the drink hot or cold.

Nutrition: Calories 523 Carbohydrates: 4.6g Protein: 47.9g Fat: 34.8g

Banana Weight Loss Juice

Preparation Time: 10 Minutes

Cooking Time: 0 Minutes

Servings: 1

Ingredients:

- Water (1/3 C.)
- Apple (1, Sliced)
- Orange (1, Sliced)
- Banana (1, Sliced)
- Lemon Juice (1 T.)

Directions:

1. Looking to boost your weight loss? The key is taking in less calories; this recipe can get you there.

2. Simply place everything into your blender, blend on high for twenty seconds, and then pour into your glass.

Nutrition: Calories: 289 Total Carbohydrate: 2 g Cholesterol: 3 mg Total Fat: 17 g Fiber: 2 g Protein: 7 g Sodium: 163 mg

Citrus Detox Juice

Preparation Time: 10 Minutes

Cooking Time: 0 Minutes

Servings: 4

Ingredients:

- Water (3 C.)
- Lemon (1, Sliced)
- Grapefruit (1, Sliced)
- Orange (1, Sliced)

Directions:

1. While starting your new diet, it is going to be vital to stay hydrated. This detox juice is the perfect solution and offers some extra flavor.

2. Begin by peeling and slicing up your fruit. Once this is done, place in a pitcher of water and infuse the water overnight.

Nutrition: Calories: 269 Total Carbohydrate: 2 g Cholesterol: 3 mg Total Fat: 14 g Fiber: 2 g Protein: 7 g Sodium: 183 mg

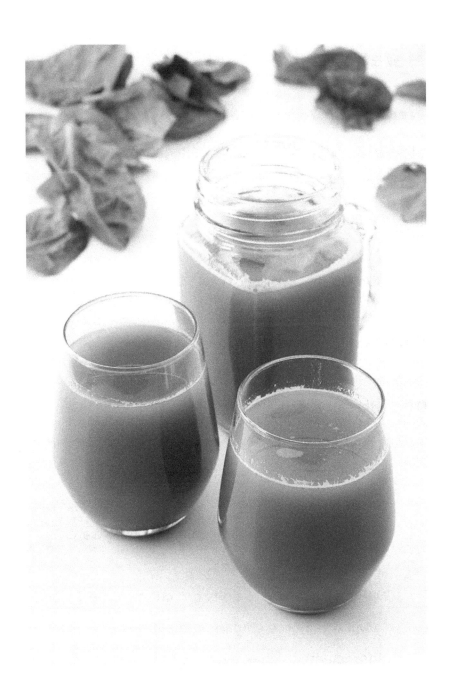

Metabolism Water

Preparation Time: 10 Minutes

Cooking Time: 0 Minutes

Servings: 1

Ingredients:

- Water (3 C.)
- Cucumber (1, Sliced)
- Lemon (1, Sliced)
- Mint (2 Leaves)
- Ice

Directions:

1. At some point, we probably all wish for a quicker metabolism! With the lemon acting as an energizer, cucumber for a refreshing taste, and mint to help your stomach digest, this water is perfect!

2. All you will have to do is get out a pitcher, place all of the ingredients in, and allow the ingredients to soak overnight for maximum benefits!

Nutrition: Calories: 301 Total Carbohydrate: 2 g
Cholesterol: 13 mg Total Fat: 17 g Fiber: 4 g
Protein: 8 g Sodium: 201 mg

Stress Relief Detox Drink

Preparation Time: 5 Minutes

Cooking Time: 0 Minutes

Servings: 1

Ingredients:

- Water (1 Pitcher)
- Mint
- Lemon (1, Sliced)
- Basil
- Strawberries (1 C., Sliced)
- Ice

Directions:

1. Life can be a pretty stressful event. Luckily, there is water to help keep you cool, calm, and collected! The lemon works like an energizer, the basil is a natural antidepressant, and mint can help your stomach do its job better. As for the strawberries, those are just for some sweetness!

2. When you are ready, take all of the ingredients and place into a pitcher of water overnight and enjoy the next day.

Nutrition: Calories: 189 Total Carbohydrate: 2 g

Cholesterol: 73 mg Total Fat: 17 g Fiber: 0 g

Protein: 7 g Sodium: 163 mg

Strawberry Pink Drink

Preparation Time: 10 Minutes

Cooking Time: 5 Minutes

Servings: 4

Ingredients:

- Water (1 C., Boiling)
- Sugar (2 T.)
- Acai Tea Bag (1)
- Coconut Milk (1 C.)
- Frozen Strawberries (1/2 C.)

Directions:

1. If you are looking for a little treat, this is going to be the recipe for you! You will begin by boiling your cup of water and seep the tea bag in for at least five minutes.

2. When the tea is set, add in the sugar and coconut milk. Be sure to stir well to spread the sweetness throughout the tea.

3. Finally, add in your strawberries, and you can enjoy your freshly made pink drink!

Nutrition: Calories: 321 Total Carbohydrate: 2 g

Cholesterol: 13 mg Total Fat: 17 g Fiber: 2 g

Protein: 9 g Sodium: 312 mg

Avocado Pudding

Preparation Time: 10 minutes

Cooking Time: 0 minute

Servings: 8

Ingredients:

- 2 ripe avocados, peeled, pitted and cut into pieces
- 1 tbsp. fresh lime juice
- 14 oz. can coconut milk
- 80 drops of liquid stevia
- 2 tsp vanilla extract

Directions:

1. Add all ingredients into the blender and blend until smooth.
2. Serve and enjoy.

Nutrition: Calories: 209 Total Carbohydrate: 6 g Cholesterol: 13 mg Total Fat: 7 g Fiber: 2 g Protein: 17 g Sodium: 193 mg

Almond Butter Brownies

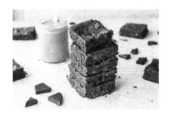

Preparation Time: 10 minutes

Cooking Time: 20 minutes

Servings: 4

Ingredients:

- 1 scoop protein powder
- 2 tbsp. cocoa powder
- 1/2 cup almond butter, melted
- 1 cup bananas, overripe

Directions:

1. Preheat the oven to 350 F/ 176 C.
1. Spray brownie tray with cooking spray.
2. Add all ingredients into the blender and blend until smooth.
3. Pour batter into the prepared dish and bake in preheated oven for 20 minutes.
4. Serve and enjoy.

Nutrition: Calories: 214 Total Carbohydrate: 2 g

Cholesterol: 73 mg Total Fat: 7 g Fiber: 2g

Protein: 19 g Sodium: 308 g

Raspberry Chia Pudding

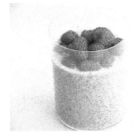

Preparation Time: 3 hours 10 minutes

Cooking Time: 0 minute

Servings: 2

Ingredients:

- 4 tbsp. chia seeds
- 1 cup coconut milk
- 1/2 cup raspberries

Directions:

1. Add raspberry and coconut milk in a blender and blend until smooth.
2. Pour mixture into the Mason jar.
3. Add chia seeds in a jar and stir well.
4. Close jar tightly with lid and shake well.
5. Place in refrigerator for 3 hours.
6. Serve chilled and enjoy.

Nutrition: Calories: 189 Total Carbohydrate: 6 g Cholesterol: 3 mg Total Fat: 7 g Fiber: 4 g Protein: 12 g Sodium: 293 mg

Chocolate Fudge

Preparation Time: 10 minutes

Cooking Time: 0 minute

Servings: 12

Ingredients:

- 4 oz. unsweetened dark chocolate
- 3/4 cup coconut butter
- 15 drops liquid stevia
- 1 tsp vanilla extract

Directions:

1. Melt coconut butter and dark chocolate.
2. Add ingredients to the large bowl and combine well.
3. Pour mixture into a silicone loaf pan and place in refrigerator until set.
4. Cut into pieces and serve.

Nutrition: Calories: 283 Total Carbohydrate: 10 g Cholesterol: 3 mg Total Fat: 8 g Fiber: 2 g Protein: 9 g Sodium: 271 mg

Quick Chocó Brownie

Preparation Time: 10 minutes

Cooking Time: 2 minutes

Servings: 1

Ingredients:

- 1/4 cup almond milk
- 1 tbsp. cocoa powder
- 1 scoop chocolate protein powder
- 1/2 tsp baking powder

Directions:

1. In a microwave-safe mug blend together baking powder, protein powder, and cocoa.
2. Add almond milk in a mug and stir well.
3. Place mug in microwave and microwave for 30 seconds.
4. Serve and enjoy.

Nutrition: Calories: 231 Total Carbohydrate: 2 g Cholesterol: 13 mg Total Fat: 15 g Fiber: 2 g Protein: 8 g Sodium: 298 mg

Simple Almond Butter Fudge

Preparation Time: 15 minutes

Cooking Time: 0 minutes

Servings: 8

Ingredients:

- 1/2 cup almond butter
- 15 drops liquid stevia
- 2 1/2 tbsp. coconut oil

Directions:

1. Combine together almond butter and coconut oil in a saucepan. Gently warm until melted.
2. Add stevia and stir well.
3. Pour mixture into the candy container and place in refrigerator until set.
4. Serve and enjoy.

Nutrition: Calories: 198 Total Carbohydrate: 5 g Cholesterol: 12 mg Total Fat: 10 g Fiber: 2 g Protein: 6 g Sodium: 257 mg

Coconut Peanut Butter Fudge

Preparation Time: 1 hour 15 minutes

Cooking Time: 0 minute

Servings: 20

Ingredients:

- 12 oz. smooth peanut butter
- 3 tbsp. coconut oil
- 4 tbsp. coconut cream
- 15 drops liquid stevia
- Pinch of salt

Directions:

1. Line baking tray with parchment paper.
2. Melt coconut oil in a saucepan over low heat.
3. Add peanut butter, coconut cream, stevia, and salt in a saucepan. Stir well.
4. Pour fudge mixture into the prepared baking tray and place in refrigerator for 1 hour.
5. Cut into pieces and serve.

Nutrition: Calories: 189 Total Carbohydrate: 2 g Cholesterol: 13 mg Total Fat: 7 g Fiber: 2 g Protein: 10 g Sodium: 301 mg

Lemon Mousse

Preparation Time: 10 minutes

Cooking Time: 0 minute

Servings: 2

Ingredients:

- 14 oz. coconut milk
- 12 drops liquid stevia
- 1/2 tsp lemon extract
- 1/4 tsp turmeric

Directions:

1. Place coconut milk can in the refrigerator for overnight. Scoop out thick cream into a mixing bowl.
2. Add remaining ingredients to the bowl and whip using a hand mixer until smooth.
3. Transfer mousse mixture to a zip-lock bag and pipe into small serving glasses. Place in refrigerator.
4. Serve chilled and enjoy.

Nutrition: Calories: 189 Total Carbohydrate: 2 g
Cholesterol: 13 mg Total Fat: 7 g Fiber: 2 g
Protein: 15 g Sodium: 321 mg

Chocó Chia Pudding

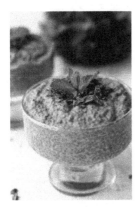

Preparation Time: 10 minutes

Cooking Time: 0 minutes

Servings: 6

Ingredients:

- 2 1/2 cups coconut milk
- 2 scoops stevia extract powder
- 6 tbsp. cocoa powder
- 1/2 cup chia seeds
- 1/2 tsp vanilla extract
- 1/8 cup xylitol
- 1/8 tsp salt

Directions:

1. Add all ingredients into the blender and blend until smooth.

2. Pour mixture into the glass container and place in refrigerator.

3. Serve chilled and enjoy.

Nutrition: Calories: 178 Total Carbohydrate: 3 g

Cholesterol: 3 mg Total Fat: 17 g Fiber: g

Protein: 9 g Sodium: 297 mg

Spiced Buttermilk

Preparation Time: 5 minutes

Cooking Time: 0 minute

Servings: 2

Ingredients:

- 3/4 teaspoon ground cumin
- 1/4 teaspoon sea salt
- 1/8 teaspoon ground black pepper
- 2 mint leaves
- 1/8 teaspoon lemon juice
- ¼ cup cilantro leaves
- 1 cup of chilled water
- 1 cup vegan yogurt, unsweetened
- Ice as needed

Directions:

1. Place all the ingredients in the order in a food processor or blender, except for cilantro and ¼ teaspoon cumin, and then pulse for 2 to 3 minutes at high speed until smooth.
2. Pour the milk into glasses, top with cilantro and cumin, and then serve.

Nutrition: Calories: 211 Total Carbohydrate: 7 g

Cholesterol: 13 mg Total Fat: 18 g Fiber: 3 g

Protein: 17 g Sodium: 289 mg

Soothing Ginger Tea Drink

Preparation Time: 5 minutes

Cooking Time: 2 hours 20 minutes

Servings: 8

Ingredients:

- 1 tablespoon of minced gingerroot
- 2 tablespoons of honey
- 15 green tea bags
- 32 fluid ounce of white grape juice
- 2 quarts of boiling water

Directions:

1. Pour water into a 4-quarts slow cooker, immerse tea bags, cover the cooker and let stand for 10 minutes.

2. After 10 minutes, remove and discard tea bags and stir in remaining ingredients.

3. Return cover to slow cooker, then plug in and let cook at high heat setting for 2 hours or until heated through.

4. When done, strain the liquid and serve hot or cold.

Nutrition: Calories 232 Carbs: 7.9g Protein: 15.9g Fat: 15.1g

Nice Spiced Cherry Cider

Preparation Time: 1 hour 5 minutes

Cooking Time: 3 hours

Servings: 16

Ingredients:

- 2 cinnamon sticks, each about 3 inches long
- 6-ounce of cherry gelatin
- 4 quarts of apple cider

Directions:

1. Using a 6-quarts slow cooker, pour the apple cider and add the cinnamon stick.
2. Stir, then cover the slow cooker with its lid. Plug in the cooker and let it cook for 3 hours at the high heat setting or until it is heated thoroughly.
3. Then add and stir the gelatin properly, then continue cooking for another hour.
4. When done, remove the cinnamon sticks and serve the drink hot or cold.

Nutrition: Calories 78 Carbs: 13.2g Protein: 2.8g Fat: 1.5g

Fragrant Spiced Coffee

Preparation Time: 10 minutes

Cooking Time: 3 hours

Servings: 8

Ingredients:

- 4 cinnamon sticks, each about 3 inches long
- 1 1/2 teaspoons of whole cloves
- 1/3 cup of honey
- 2-ounce of chocolate syrup
- 1/2 teaspoon of anise extract
- 8 cups of brewed coffee

Directions:

1. Pour the coffee in a 4-quarts slow cooker and pour in the remaining ingredients except for cinnamon and stir properly.

2. Wrap the whole cloves in cheesecloth and tie its corners with strings.

3. Immerse this cheesecloth bag in the liquid present in the slow cooker and cover it with the lid.

4. Then plug in the slow cooker and let it cook on the low heat setting for 3 hours or until heated thoroughly.

5. When done, discard the cheesecloth bag and serve.

Nutrition: Calories 136 Fat 12.6 g Carbohydrates 4.1 g Sugar 0.5 g Protein 10.3 g Cholesterol 88 mg

Bracing Coffee Smoothie

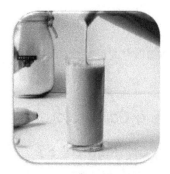

Preparation Time: 5 minutes

Cooking Time: 5 minutes

Servings: 1

Ingredients:

- 1 banana, sliced and frozen
- ½ cup strong brewed coffee
- ½ cup milk
- ¼ cup rolled oats
- 1 tsp nut butter

Directions:

1. Mix all the ingredients until smooth.
2. Enjoy your morning drink!

Nutrition: Calories 414 Fat 20.6 g Carbohydrates 5.6 g Sugar 1.3 g Protein 48.8 g Cholesterol 58 mg

Vitamin Green Smoothie

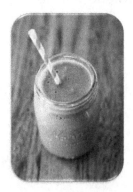

Preparation Time: 5 minutes

Cooking Time: 5 minutes

Servings: 2

Ingredients:

- 1 cup milk or juice
- 1 cup spinach or kale
- ½ cup plain yoghurt
- 1 kiwi
- 1 Tbsp. chia or flax
- 1 tsp vanilla

Directions:

1. Mix the milk or juice and greens until smooth. Add the remaining ingredients and continue blending until smooth again.

2. Enjoy your delicious drink!

Nutrition: Calories 397 Fat 36.4 g Carbohydrates 4 g Sugar 1 g Protein 14.7 g Cholesterol 4 mg

Strawberry Grapefruit Smoothie

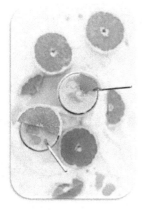

Preparation Time: 5 minutes

Cooking Time: 5 minutes

Servings: 2

Ingredients:

- 1 banana

- ½ cup strawberries, frozen

- 1 grapefruit

- ¼ cup milk

- ¼ cup plain yoghurt

- 2 Tbsp. honey

- ½ tsp ginger, chopped

Directions:

1. Using a mixer, blend all the ingredients.

2. When smooth, top your drink with a slice of grapefruit and enjoy it!

Nutrition: Calories 233 Fat 7.9 g Carbohydrates 3.2 g Sugar 0.1 g Protein 35.6 g Cholesterol 32 m

Inspirational Orange Smoothie

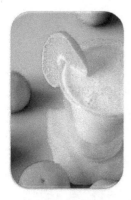

Preparation Time: 5 minutes

Cooking Time: 5 minutes

Servings: 1

Ingredients:

- 4 mandarin oranges, peeled
- 1 banana, sliced and frozen
- ½ cup non-fat Greek yoghurt
- ¼ cup coconut water
- 1 tsp vanilla extract
- 5 ice cubes

Directions:

1. Using a mixer, whisk all the ingredients.
2. Enjoy your drink!

Nutrition: Calories 256 Fat 13.3 g Carbohydrates 0 g Sugar 0 g Protein 34.5 g Cholesterol 78 mg

High Protein Blueberry Banana Smoothie

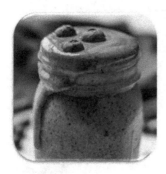

Preparation Time: 5 minutes

Cooking Time: 5 minutes

Servings: 2

Ingredients:

- 1 cup blueberries, frozen
- 2 ripe bananas
- 1 cup water
- 1 tsp vanilla extract
- 2 Tbsp. chia seeds
- ½ cup cottage cheese
- 1 tsp lemon zest

Directions:

1. Put all the smoothie ingredients into the blender and whisk until smooth.

2. Enjoy your wonderful smoothie!

Nutrition: Calories 358 Fat 19.8 g Carbohydrates 1.3 g Sugar 0.4 g Protein 41.9 g Cholesterol 131 mg

Ginger Smoothie with Citrus and Mint

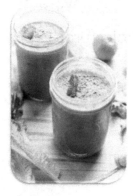

Preparation Time: 5 minutes

Cooking Time: 3 minutes

Servings: 3

Ingredients:

- 1 head Romaine lettuce, chopped into 4 chunks
- 2 Tbsp. hemp seeds
- 5 mandarin oranges, peeled
- 1 banana, frozen
- 1 carrot
- 2-3 mint leaves
- ½ piece ginger root, peeled
- 1 cup water

- ¼ lemon, peeled
- ½ cup ice

Directions:

1. Put all the smoothie ingredients in a blender and blend until smooth.
2. Enjoy!

Nutrition: Calories 101 Fat 4 g Carbohydrates 14 g Sugar 1 g Protein 2 g Cholesterol 3 mg

Strawberry Beet Smoothie

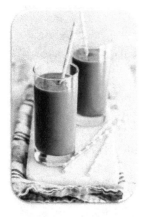

Preparation Time: 5 minutes

Cooking Time: 50 minutes

Servings: 2

Ingredients:

- 1 red beet, trimmed, peeled and chopped into cubes
- 1 cup strawberries, quartered
- 1 ripe banana
- ½ cup strawberry yoghurt
- 1 Tbsp. honey
- 1 Tbsp. water
- Milk, to taste

Directions:

1. Sprinkle the beet cubes with water, place on aluminum foil and put in the oven (preheated to 204°C). Bake for 40 minutes.
2. Let the baked beet cool.
3. Combine all the smoothie ingredients.
4. Enjoy your fantastic drink.

Nutrition: Calories 184 Fat 9.2 g Carbohydrates 1 g Sugar 0.4 g Protein 24.9 g Cholesterol 132 mg

Peanut Butter Shake

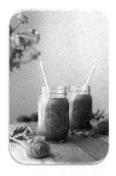

Preparation Time: 5 minutes

Cooking Time: 5 minutes

Servings: 2

Ingredients:

- 1 cup plant-based milk
- 1 handful kale
- 2 bananas, frozen
- 2 Tbsp. peanut butter
- ½ tsp ground cinnamon
- ¼ tsp vanilla powder

Directions:

1. Use a blender to combine all the ingredients for your shake.
2. Enjoy it!

Nutrition: Calories 184 Fat 9.2 g Carbohydrates 1 g Sugar 0.4 g Protein 24.9 g Cholesterol 132 mg

DESSERTS

Chocolate and Avocado Pudding

Preparation Time: 3 hours and 10 minutes

Cooking Time: 0 minute

Servings: 1

Ingredients:

- 1 small avocado, pitted, peeled
- 1 small banana, mashed
- 1/3 cup cocoa powder, unsweetened
- 1 tablespoon cacao nibs, unsweetened
- 1/4 cup maple syrup
- 1/3 cup coconut cream

Directions:

1. Add avocado in a food processor along with cream and then pulse for 2 minutes until smooth.

2. Add remaining ingredients, blend until mixed, and then tip the pudding in a container.

3. Cover the container with a plastic wrap; it should touch the pudding and refrigerate for 3 hours.

4. Serve straight away.

Nutrition: Calories: 87 Cal Fat: 7 g Carbs: 9 g Protein: 1.5 g Fiber: 3.2 g

Chocolate Avocado Ice Cream

Preparation Time: 1 hour and 10 minutes

Cooking Time: 0 minute

Servings: 2

Ingredients:

- 4.5 ounces avocado, peeled, pitted
- 1/2 cup cocoa powder, unsweetened
- 1 tablespoon vanilla extract, unsweetened
- 1/2 cup and 2 tablespoons maple syrup
- 13.5 ounces coconut milk, unsweetened
- 1/2 cup water

Directions:

1. Add avocado in a food processor along with milk and then pulse for 2 minutes until smooth.
2. Add remaining ingredients, blend until mixed, and then tip the pudding in a freezer-proof container.
3. Place the container in a freezer and chill for freeze for 4 hours until firm, whisking every 20 minutes after 1 hour.
4. Serve straight away.

Nutrition: Calories: 80.7 Cal Fat: 7.1 g Carbs: 6

g Protein: 0.6 g Fiber: 2 g

Watermelon Mint Popsicles

Preparation Time: 8 hours and 5 minutes

Cooking Time: 0 minute

Servings: 8

Ingredients:

- 20 mint leaves, diced
- 6 cups watermelon chunks
- 3 tablespoons lime juice

Directions:

1. Add watermelon in a food processor along with lime juice and then pulse for 15 seconds until smooth.

2. Pass the watermelon mixture through a strainer placed over a bowl, remove the seeds and then stir mint into the collected watermelon mixture.

3. Take eight Popsicle molds, pour in prepared watermelon mixture, and freeze for 2 hours until slightly firm.

4. Then insert popsicle sticks and continue freezing for 6 hours until solid.

5. Serve straight away

Nutrition: Calories: 90 Cal Fat: 0 g Carbs: 23 g

Protein: 0 g Fiber: 0 g

Mango Coconut Chia Pudding

Preparation Time: 2 hours and 5 minutes

Cooking Time: 0 minute

Servings: 1

Ingredients:

- 1 medium mango, peeled, cubed
- 1/4 cup chia seeds
- 2 tablespoons coconut flakes
- 1 cup coconut milk, unsweetened
- 1 1/2 teaspoons maple syrup

Directions:

1. Take a bowl, place chia seeds in it, whisk in milk until combined, and then stir in maple syrup.

2. Cover the bowl with a plastic wrap; it should touch the pudding mixture and refrigerate for 2 hours until the pudding has set.

3. Then puree mango until smooth, top it evenly over pudding, sprinkle with coconut flakes and serve.

Nutrition: Calories: 159 Cal Fat: 9 g Carbs: 17 g Protein: 3 g Fiber: 6 g

Brownie Energy Bites

Preparation Time: 1 hour and 10 minutes

Cooking Time: 0 minute

Servings: 2

Ingredients:

- 1/2 cup walnuts
- 1 cup Medjool dates, chopped
- 1/2 cup almonds
- 1/8 teaspoon salt
- 1/2 cup shredded coconut flakes
- 1/3 cup and 2 teaspoons cocoa powder, unsweetened

Directions:

1. Place almonds and walnuts in a food processor and pulse for 3 minutes until the dough starts to come together.
2. Add remaining ingredients, reserving ¼ cup of coconut and pulse for 2 minutes until incorporated.

3. Shape the mixture into balls, roll them in remaining coconut until coated, and refrigerate for 1 hour.

4. Serve straight away

Nutrition: Calories: 174.6 Cal Fat: 8.1 g Carbs: 25.5 g Protein: 4.1 g Fiber: 4.4 g

Strawberry Coconut Ice Cream

Preparation Time: 5 minutes

Cooking Time: 0 minute

Servings: 4

Ingredients:

- 4 cups frouncesen strawberries
- 1 vanilla bean, seeded
- 28 ounces coconut cream
- 1/2 cup maple syrup

Directions:

1. Place cream in a food processor and pulse for 1 minute until soft peaks come together.
2. Then tip the cream in a bowl, add remaining ingredients in the blender and blend until thick mixture comes together.
3. Add the mixture into the cream, fold until combined, and then transfer ice cream into a freezer-safe bowl and freeze for 4 hours until firm, whisking every 20 minutes after 1 hour.
4. Serve straight away.

Nutrition: Calories: 100 Cal Fat: 100 g Carbs: 100 g Protein: 100 g Fiber: 100 g

Salted Caramel Chocolate Cups

Preparation Time: 5 minutes

Cooking Time: 2 minutes

Servings: 12

Ingredients:

- ¼ teaspoon sea salt granules

- 1 cup dark chocolate chips, unsweetened

- 2 teaspoons coconut oil

- 6 tablespoons caramel sauce

Directions:

1. Take a heatproof bowl, add chocolate chips and oil, stir until mixed, then microwave for 1 minute until melted, stir chocolate and continue heating in the microwave for 30 seconds.

2. Take twelve mini muffin tins, line them with muffin liners, spoon a little bit of chocolate mixture into the tins, spread the chocolate in the bottom and along the sides, and freeze for 10 minutes until set.

3. Then fill each cup with ½ tablespoon of caramel sauce, cover with remaining chocolate and freeze for another 2salt0 minutes until set.

4. When ready to eat, peel off liner from the cup, sprinkle with sauce, and serve.

Nutrition: Calories: 80 Cal Fat: 5 g Carbs: 10 g Protein: 1 g Fiber: 0.5 g

Chocolate Peanut Butter Energy Bites

Preparation Time: 1 hour and 5 minutes

Cooking Time: 0 minute

Servings: 4

Ingredients:

- 1/2 cup oats, old-fashioned
- 1/3 cup cocoa powder, unsweetened
- 1 cup dates, chopped
- 1/2 cup shredded coconut flakes, unsweetened
- 1/2 cup peanut butter

Directions:

1. Place oats in a food processor along with dates and pulse for 1 minute until the paste starts to come together.
2. Then add remaining ingredients, and blend until incorporated and very thick mixture comes together.
3. Shape the mixture into balls, refrigerate for 1 hour until set and then serve.

Nutrition: Calories: 88.6 Cal Fat: 5 g Carbs: 10 g

Protein: 2.3 g Fiber: 1.6 g

Mango Coconut Cheesecake

Preparation Time: 4 hours and 10 minutes

Cooking Time: 0 minute

Servings: 4

Ingredients:

For the Crust:

- 1 cup macadamia nuts
- 1 cup dates, pitted, soaked in hot water for 10 minutes

For the Filling:

- 2 cups cashews, soaked in warm water for 10 minutes
- 1/2 cup and 1 tablespoon maple syrup
- 1/3 cup and 2 tablespoons coconut oil
- 1/4 cup lemon juice
- 1/2 cup and 2 tablespoons coconut milk, unsweetened, chilled

For the Topping:

- 1 cup fresh mango slices

Directions:

1. Prepare the crust, and for this, place nuts in a food processor and process until mixture resembles crumbs.
2. Drain the dates, add them to the food processor and blend for 2 minutes until thick mixture comes together.
3. Take a 4-inch cheesecake pan, place date mixture in it, spread and press evenly, and set aside.
4. Prepare the filling and for this, place all its ingredients in a food processor and blend for 3 minutes until smooth.
5. Pour the filling into the crust, spread evenly, and then freeze for 4 hours until set.
6. Top the cake with mango slices and then serve.

Nutrition: Calories: 200 Cal Fat: 11 g Carbs: 22.5 g Protein: 2 g Fiber: 1 g

Rainbow Fruit Salad

Preparation Time: 10 minutes

Cooking Time: 0 minute

Servings: 4

Ingredients:

For the Fruit Salad:

- 1 pound strawberries, hulled, sliced
- 1 cup kiwis, halved, cubed
- 1 1/4 cups blueberries
- 1 1/3 cups blackberries
- 1 cup pineapple chunks

For the Maple Lime Dressing:

- 2 teaspoons lime zest
- 1/4 cup maple syrup
- 1 tablespoon lime juice

Directions:

1. Prepare the salad, and for this, take a bowl, place all its ingredients and toss until mixed.

2. Prepare the dressing, and for this, take a small bowl, place all its ingredients and whisk well.

3. Drizzle the dressing over salad, toss until coated and serve.

Nutrition: Calories: 88.1 Cal Fat: 0.4 g Carbs: 22.6 g Protein: 1.1 g Fiber: 2.8 g

Cookie Dough Bites

Preparation Time: 4 hours and 10 minutes

Cooking Time: 0 minute

Servings: 18

Ingredients:

- 15 ounces cooked chickpeas
- 1/3 cup vegan chocolate chips
- 1/3 cup and 2 tablespoons peanut butter
- 8 Medjool dates pitted
- 1 teaspoon vanilla extract, unsweetened
- 2 tablespoons maple syrup
- 1 1/2 tablespoons almond milk, unsweetened

Directions:

1. Place chickpeas in a food processor along with dates, butter, and vanilla and then process for 2 minutes until smooth.
2. Add remaining ingredients, except for chocolate chips, and then pulse for 1 minute until blends and dough comes together.

3. Add chocolate chips, stir until just mixed, and then shape the mixture into 18 balls and refrigerate for 4 hours until firm.

4. Serve straight away

Nutrition: Calories: 200 Cal Fat: 9 g Carbs: 26 g Protein: 1 g Fiber: 0 g

Dark Chocolate Bars

Preparation Time: 1 hour and 10 minutes

Cooking Time: 2 minutes

Servings: 12

Ingredients:

- 1 cup cocoa powder, unsweetened
- 3 Tablespoons cacao nibs
- 1/8 teaspoon sea salt
- 2 Tablespoons maple syrup
- 1 1/4 cup chopped cocoa butter
- 1/2 teaspoons vanilla extract, unsweetened
- 2 Tablespoons coconut oil

Directions:

1. Take a heatproof bowl, add butter, oil, stir, and microwave for 90 to 120 seconds until melts, stirring every 30 seconds.
2. Sift cocoa powder over melted butter mixture, whisk well until combined, and then stir in maple syrup, vanilla, and salt until mixed.

3. Distribute the mixture evenly between twelve mini cupcake liners, top with cacao nibs, and freeze for 1 hour until set.

4. Serve straight away

Nutrition: Calories: 100 Cal Fat: 9 g Carbs: 8 g Protein: 2 g Fiber: 2 g

Almond Butter, Oat and Protein Energy Balls

Preparation Time: 1 hour and 10 minutes

Cooking Time: 3 minutes

Servings: 4

Ingredients:

- 1 cup rolled oats
- ½ cup honey
- 2 ½ scoops of vanilla protein powder
- 1 cup almond butter
- Chia seeds for rolling

Directions:

1. Take a skillet pan, place it over medium heat, add butter and honey, stir and cook for 2 minutes until warm.
2. Transfer the mixture into a bowl, stir in protein powder until mixed, and then stir in oatmeal until combined.

3. Shape the mixture into balls, roll them into chia seeds, then arrange them on a cookie sheet and refrigerate for 1 hour until firm.

4. Serve straight away

Nutrition: Calories: 200 Cal Fat: 10 g Carbs: 21 g Protein: 7 g Fiber: 4 g

Chocolate and Avocado Truffles

Preparation Time: 1 hour and 10 minutes

Cooking Time: 1 minute

Servings: 18

Ingredients:

- 1 medium avocado, ripe
- 2 tablespoons cocoa powder
- 10 ounces of dark chocolate chips

Directions:

1. Scoop out the flesh from avocado, place it in a bowl, then mash with a fork until smooth, and stir in 1/2 cup chocolate chips.

2. Place remaining chocolate chips in a heatproof bowl and microwave for 1 minute until chocolate has melted, stirring halfway.

3. Add melted chocolate into avocado mixture, stir well until blended, and then refrigerate for 1 hour.

4. Then shape the mixture into balls, 1 tablespoon of mixture per ball, and roll in cocoa powder until covered.

5. Serve straight away.

Nutrition: Calories: 59 Cal Fat: 4 g Carbs: 7 g

Protein: 0 g Fiber: 1 g

Coconut Oil Cookies

Preparation Time: 10 minutes

Cooking Time: 10 minutes

Servings: 15

Ingredients:

- 3 1/4 cup oats
- 1/2 teaspoons salt
- 2 cups coconut Sugar
- 1 teaspoons vanilla extract, unsweetened
- 1/4 cup cocoa powder
- 1/2 cup liquid Coconut Oil
- 1/2 cup peanut butter
- 1/2 cup cashew milk

Directions:

1. Take a saucepan, place it over medium heat, add all the ingredients except for oats and vanilla, stir until mixed, and then bring the mixture to boil.

2. Simmer the mixture for 4 minutes, mixing frequently, then remove the pan from heat and stir in vanilla.

3. Add oats, stir until well mixed and then scoop the mixture on a plate lined with wax paper.

4. Serve straight away.

Nutrition: Calories: 112 Cal Fat: 6.5 g Carbs: 13 g Protein: 1.4 g Fiber: 0.1 g

Apple Crumble

Preparation Time: 20 minutes

Cooking Time: 25 minutes

Servings: 6

Ingredients:

- For the filling
- 4 to 5 apples, cored and chopped (about 6 cups)
- ½ cup unsweetened applesauce, or ¼ cup water
- 2 to 3 tablespoons unrefined sugar (coconut, date, sucanat, maple syrup)
- 1 teaspoon ground cinnamon
- Pinch sea salt
- For the crumble
- 2 tablespoons almond butter, or cashew or sunflower seed butter
- 2 tablespoons maple syrup
- 1½ cups rolled oats
- ½ cup walnuts, finely chopped
- ½ teaspoon ground cinnamon
- 2 to 3 tablespoons unrefined granular sugar (coconut, date, sucanat)

Directions:

1. Preparing the Ingredients.

2. Preheat the oven to 350°F. Put the apples and applesauce in an 8-inch-square baking dish, and sprinkle with the sugar, cinnamon, and salt. Toss to combine.

3. In a medium bowl, mix together the nut butter and maple syrup until smooth and creamy. Add the oats, walnuts, cinnamon, and sugar and stir to coat, using your hands if necessary. (If you have a small food processor, pulse the oats and walnuts together before adding them to the mix.)

4. Sprinkle the topping over the apples, and put the dish in the oven.

5. Bake for 20 to 25 minutes, or until the fruit is soft and the topping is lightly browned.

Nutrition: Calories 195 Fat 7 g Carbohydrates 6 g Sugar 2 g Protein 24 g Cholesterol 65 mg

Cashew-Chocolate Truffles

Preparation Time: 15 minutes

Cooking Time: 0 minutes

Servings: 12

Ingredients:

- 1 cup raw cashews, soaked in water overnight
- ¾ cup pitted dates
- 2 tablespoons coconut oil
- 1 cup unsweetened shredded coconut, divided
- 1 to 2 tablespoons cocoa powder, to taste

Directions:

1. Preparing the Ingredients.

2. In a food processor, combine the cashews, dates, coconut oil, ½ cup of shredded coconut, and cocoa powder. Pulse until fully incorporated; it will resemble chunky cookie dough. Spread the remaining ½ cup of shredded coconut on a plate.

3. Form the mixture into tablespoon-size balls and roll on the plate to cover with the shredded coconut. Transfer to a parchment paper–lined

plate or baking sheet. Repeat to make 12 truffles.

4. Place the truffles in the refrigerator for 1 hour to set. Transfer the truffles to a storage container or freezer-safe bag and seal.

Nutrition: Calories 160 Fat 1 g Carbohydrates 1 g Sugar 0.5 g Protein 22 g Cholesterol 60 mg

Banana Chocolate Cupcakes

Preparation Time: 20 minutes

Cooking Time: 20 minutes

Servings: 1

Ingredients:

- 3 medium bananas
- 1 cup non-dairy milk
- 2 tablespoons almond butter
- 1 teaspoon apple cider vinegar
- 1 teaspoon pure vanilla extract
- 1¼ cups whole-grain flour
- ½ cup rolled oats
- ¼ cup coconut sugar (optional)
- 1 teaspoon baking powder
- ½ teaspoon baking soda
- ½ cup unsweetened cocoa powder
- ¼ cup chia seeds, or sesame seeds
- Pinch sea salt
- ¼ cup dark chocolate chips, dried cranberries, or raisins (optional)

Directions:

1. Preparing the Ingredients.

2. Preheat the oven to 350°F. Lightly grease the cups of two 6-cup muffin tins or line with paper muffin cups.

3. Put the bananas, milk, almond butter, vinegar, and vanilla in a blender and purée until smooth. Or stir together in a large bowl until smooth and creamy.

4. Put the flour, oats, sugar (if using), baking powder, baking soda, cocoa powder, chia seeds, salt, and chocolate chips in another large bowl, and stir to combine. Mix together the wet and dry ingredients, stirring as little as possible. Spoon into muffin cups, and bake for 20 to 25 minutes. Take the cupcakes out of the oven and let them cool fully before taking out of the muffin tins, since they'll be very moist.

Nutrition: Calories 295 Fat 17 g Carbohydrates 4 g Sugar 0.1 g Protein 29 g Cholesterol 260 mg

Minty Fruit Salad

Preparation Time: 15 minutes

Cooking Time: 5 minutes

Servings: 4

Ingredients:

- ¼ cup lemon juice (about 2 small lemons)
- 4 teaspoons maple syrup or agave syrup
- 2 cups chopped pineapple
- 2 cups chopped strawberries
- 2 cups raspberries
- 1 cup blueberries
- 8 fresh mint leaves

Directions:

Preparing the Ingredients.

1. Beginning with 1 mason jar, add the ingredients in this order:

2. 1 tablespoon of lemon juice, 1 teaspoon of maple syrup, ½ cup of pineapple, ½ cup of strawberries, ½ cup of raspberries, ¼ cup of blueberries, and 2 mint leaves.

3. Repeat to fill 3 more jars. Close the jars tightly with lids.

4. Place the airtight jars in the refrigerator for up to 3 days.

Nutrition: Calories 339 Fat 17.5 g Carbohydrates 2 g Sugar 2 g Protein 44 g Cholesterol 100 mg

Mango Coconut Cream Pie

Preparation Time: 20 minutes

Cooking Time: 30 minutes

Servings: 8

Ingredients:

- For the crust
- ½ cup rolled oats
- 1 cup cashews
- 1 cup soft pitted dates
- For the filling
- 1 cup canned coconut milk
- ½ cup water
- 2 large mangos, peeled and chopped, or about 2 cups frozen chunks
- ½ cup unsweetened shredded coconut

Directions:

1. Preparing the Ingredients.
2. Put all the crust ingredients in a food processor and pulse until it holds together. If you don't have a food processor, chop everything as finely as possible and use ½ cup cashew or almond

butter in place of half the cashews. Press the mixture down firmly into an 8-inch pie or springform pan.

3. Put the all filling ingredients in a blender and purée until smooth (about 1 minute). It should be very thick, so you may have to stop and stir until it's smooth.

4. Pour the filling into the crust, use a rubber spatula to smooth the top, and put the pie in the freezer until set, about 30 minutes. Once frozen, it should be set out for about 15 minutes to soften before serving.

5. Top with a batch of Coconut Whipped Cream scooped on top of the pie once it's set. Finish it off with a sprinkling of toasted shredded coconut.

Nutrition: Calories 545 Fat 39.6 g Carbohydrates 9.5 g Sugar 3.1 g Protein 43 g Cholesterol 110 mg

Cherry-Vanilla Rice Pudding (Pressure cooker)

Preparation Time: 5 minutes

Cooking Time: 30 minutes

Servings: 4-6

Ingredients:

- 1 cup short-grain brown rice
- 1¾ cups nondairy milk, plus more as needed
- 1½ cups water
- 4 tablespoons unrefined sugar or pure maple syrup (use 2 tablespoons if you use a sweetened milk), plus more as needed
- 1 teaspoon vanilla extract (use ½ teaspoon if you use vanilla milk)
- Pinch salt
- ¼ cup dried cherries or ½ cup fresh or frozen pitted cherries

Directions:

1. Preparing the Ingredients. In your electric pressure cooker's cooking pot, combine the rice, milk, water, sugar, vanilla, and salt.

2. High pressure for 30 minutes. Close and lock the lid, and select High Pressure for 30 minutes.

3. Pressure Release. Once the **Cooking Time:** is complete, let the pressure release naturally, about 20 minutes. Unlock and remove the lid. Stir in the cherries and put the lid back on loosely for about 10 minutes. Serve, adding more milk or sugar, as desired.

Nutrition: Calories 420 Fat 27.4 g Carbohydrates 2 g Sugar 0.3 g Protein 46.3 g Cholesterol 98 mg

Conclusion

Vegan recipes do not need to be boring. There are so many different combinations of veggies, fruits, whole grains, beans, seeds, and nuts that you will be able to make unique meal plans for many months. These recipes contain the instructions along with the necessary ingredients and nutritional information.

If you ever come across someone complaining that they can't follow the plant-based diet because it's expensive, hard to cater for, lacking in variety, or tasteless, feel free to have them take a look at this book. In no time, you'll have another companion walking beside you on this road to healthier eating and better living.

Although healthy, many people are still hesitant to give vegan food a try. They mistakenly believe that these would be boring, tasteless, and complicated to make. This is the farthest thing from the truth.

Fruits and vegetables are organically delicious, fragrant, and vibrantly colored. If you add herbs, mushrooms, and nuts to the mix, dishes will always come out packed full of flavor it only takes a bit of effort and time to prepare great-tasting vegan meals for your family.

How easy was that? Don't we all want a seamless and easy way to cook like this?

I believe cooking is taking a better turn and the days, when we needed so many ingredients to provide a decent meal, were gone. Now, with easy tweaks, we can make delicious, quick, and easy meals. Most importantly, we get to save a bunch of cash on groceries.

I am grateful for downloading this book and taking the time to read it. I know that you have learned a lot and you had a great time reading it. Writing books is the best way to share the skills I have with your and the best tips too.

I know that there are many books and choosing my book is amazing. I am thankful that you stopped and took time to decide. You made a great decision and I am sure that you enjoyed it.

I will be even happier if you will add some comments. Feedbacks helped by growing and they still do. They help me to choose better content and new ideas. So, maybe your feedback can trigger an idea for my next book.

Hopefully, this book has helped you understand that vegetarian recipes and diet can improve your life, not only by improving your health and helping you lose weight, but also by saving you money and time. I sincerely hope that the recipes provided in this book have proven to be quick, easy, and delicious, and have provided you with enough variety to keep your taste buds interested and curious.

I hope you enjoyed reading about my book!

CPSIA information can be obtained
at www.ICGtesting.com
Printed in the USA
BVHW091022190421
605287BV00002B/93

9 781801 835831